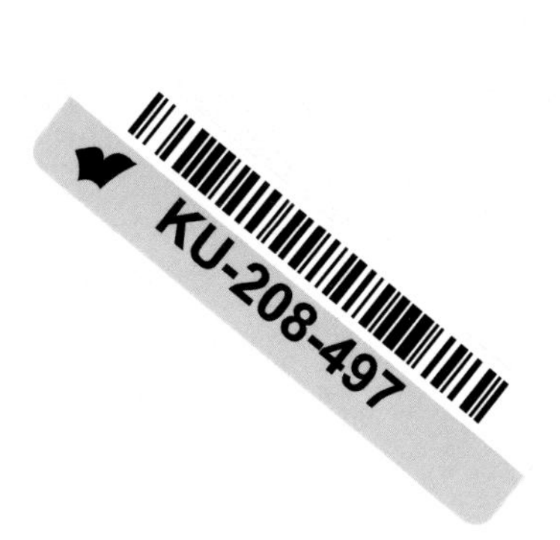

Thank you for your trust

Short Stories for Elderly

Large Print, Easy-to-Read and Short Paragraphs—
Perfect to Stimulate Memory

KIOSK 2000 PUBLISHER

INTRODUCTION

In this book you will find a short story to keep your mind busy, or a small tale to pass the time. The mind needs to be stimulated constantly in order to keep ideas fresh and your imagination active.

This book brings you 100 short stories filledwith description. It helps you think about colors,sights, sounds, tastes, smells, and feelings. Each story is designed to get you thinking and keep your imagination working.

Stimulate your memory by closing your eyesand imagine the colors of a rainbow filling the sky. Recall the salty smell of the ocean and the calming sound of the waves. Remember the smell of marshmallows roasting on a fire and the sweet, sticky taste. The sound of crickets in the tall grass is hard to forget, and the smell of rain on a hot day is easy to remember.

These experiences and many more are awaiting you in the pages ahead.

Each and every single one of these 100 stories are specially made to stimulate your memory, keep your mind active, and keep your imagination alive.

CONTENTS

100 Short Stories for Elderly

A RAINBOW IS BORN

The sky is a clear, light shade of blue. Thick, white clouds drift slowly by. The sun begins to rise over the mountains, capped by a layer of crisp, fresh snow.

A bird sings its song in the distance and the sweet sound echoes through the air. Colors spring from nothing and fill the empty sky. A still body of water holds the colors as they rise up and curve through the blue.

A rainbow is born of light, reflection, and water. The drops of water float through the air, too small to notice. They catch the light and the colors spring to life. The rainbow spreads across the sky.

It is a beautiful sight to behold and a wonder of the world. A rainbow is simply a collection of red, orange, yellow, green, blue, indigo, and violet. These colors are so wild and wonderful.

A bird sings their song and the world is filled with color for all to see.

A PEBBLE ON THE BEACH

The sounds of the beach fills your ears. The seagulls hover above your head. Their cries are heard only quietly over the wind. The waves crash onto the sand and slam into the rocks rising out of the ocean.

You feel the soft, warm sand underneath your bare feet. You walk forward, stepping into the unknown. Your feet now feel the wet sand, gently washed by the ocean's waters. With each step, you sink deeper into the sand, creating a warm blanket for your feet.

The seagulls' cries grow louder, but are still barely heard over the gusts of wind that carry a salty taste. The sun is rising. Its light reflects off the still water in the distance, past the waves.

You look down, as something cold and smooth touches your foot. It's a pebble. It's grey and flat. You reach down and save it from the waves, threatening to pull it out to sea. It feels cold in your hands and your fingers slide easily over its surface.

A pebble on the beach is a sign of luck, so you putit in your pocket and keep it safe. The sun rises into the clear blue sky. You take a deep breath. You carry the pebble home with you, keeping it close to remember you went to the beach.

CRICKETS IN THE GRASS

A cool breeze flows through the open window on a perfect spring day. The tall grass dances outside. The drops of dew catch the light and reflect it, shining like diamonds.

Today is the perfect day to sit and listen to the songs crickets sing. They lay in the tall grass, waiting for a moment to pounce. The wind blows the grass wildly. It is unsafe.

The air is silent, but not for long. The howl of the wind dies down and the crickets know it is their turn. They hop out from their hiding place. Jumping up and down in the grass, the dew drops from the tips of the grass fling about as the crickets land.

The air is soon filled with their songs. They are joined by the humming of the birds and the buzzing of the bees. It's the song of spring. They sing for all who wish to hear, and play whenever the weather is clear.

The wind returns and the crickets retreat into the grass once again. They wait for another time, to play their song once again.

RAINDROPS IN THE SUN

It's a rare sight to see: the raindrops falling through the sunlit sky. The sun shines down, warm and inviting. The thin clouds glide across the crisp, blue sky. The clouds hold a surprise only seen on dark and gloomy days.

A single drop of rain falls through the air, inviting more to follow. It catches the light, shining bright, and glints like a jewel in the sky. It sizzles on the ground, heated by the afternoon sun. The smell rises into the air. That was just the first drop of many.

The thin clouds burst into a shower of droplets. The rain falls gently. The drops are as thin as the clouds they came from. It creates not a shower, but a mist in the air. Each drop sizzling on the warm ground, like bacon frying in a pan.

The smell of rain heating up on the warm ground fills the air. Its light drumming on the tin roofs and tile walls is like music to the ears. You sit back and breathe in deep, listening to the tune.

A GOOD BOOK

A bookshelf stands against the wall at the back of the room. Beside it sits a wicker chair placed just in front of a window. The window is low enough so that you can look out into the garden while you sit back. The sun shines through the window, warming the plush pillow on the chair and providing the perfect amount of light.

On the table beside the chair is a cup of coffee. The coffee is strong and sweet, filling the room with its alluring aroma. The coffee is accompanied by a selection of small cakes and biscuits—any and all flavors you could ever want.

After a while you go through the books on the shelf, scanning the many titles, picking out one that calls to you. You sit down, sinking into the plush pillow, letting the warmth of the sun blanket you.

The book rests in your hand, its pages are crisp and smell of ink. You lift the cup of coffee from its spot on the table. Take in a deep breath and allow the coffee to wake you up, to energize you.

Lean back and open your book. The words dance on the pages, eager to tell you a story or two.

A PICNIC IN THE PARK

You're invited to a picnic in the park. The invitation arrives at your door. It's lined with gold and feels like silk. The handwriting is elegant and the words are written with a silver pen. It smells like dew-covered grass and spring water.

You arrive, and the picnic is laid out on the deep green grass. You've never seen grass so green or felt grass so soft. The blanket looks like a cloud on the ground. You sit and melt into its soft touch.

The food is laid out before you: chocolate-covered strawberries, small vanilla cakes, caramel-frosted brownies, elegant finger sandwiches, and a pot of hot tea to wash it all down. You can eat what you want and drink what you want.

The park is quiet, only the sounds of nature can be heard—the wind rustling through the autumn leaves. The squirrels chatter in the trees. The hummingbird buzzes by and the woodchucker knocksaway. A butterfly floats by and a bee buzzes along. You sit and listen to the world around you.

A LONG FLIGHT

The wind grows cold and the sun starts to set earlier in the day. When the darkness falls, the ice begins to grow. It's winter and the birds musttake flight for a new home.

They fluff up their feathers and shake out their tails. They must leave their nests behind, but they will make new ones.

The sky is still dark, but the sun begins to peek from beneath the ground. It's the first sign of light and the birds take flight. Their flight is long, but it's one they make each year. They fly away from the winter and make for the warmth of summer.

The sky is filled with birds as they travel together. They draw images in the sky of arrows pointing the way to their destination and circling the clouds in the sky. They dance among the stars and fly between the clouds.

It's a long flight and we will miss their songs, but when the sun rises early and sets late once again, we will see them return.

A PENGUIN ON A MISSION

They say when one penguin loves another penguin, they will search the entire beach for a perfect pebble to give to their partner as a present. A penguin will journey long and hard, in search of that perfect pebble.

Imagine a penguin, marching for hours and days, up and down a beach in search of one thing. There'll be thousands of pebbles on this beach, but this penguin is only interested in one.

How do they choose the perfect pebble? Do they choose it by how smooth the pebble is? Does its color come into play? Will the penguin prefer a grey pebble over a darker one? Will the penguin choose the smoothest, smallest pebble or the largest, roughest one?

How does this penguin know that the object of their affections will accept the pebble they searched for? They can only hope that the pebble they have chosen is the perfect pebble for theone they love.

THE LONELY MOUNTAIN

A mountain stands tall and mighty, alone and surrounded by a valley. The valley is full of life. Trees and flowers grow aplenty, blooming in spring and resting in autumn. Many animals call this place their home.

Deers graze in the long grass fields. Bees build their hives and harvest pollen from the flowers all around. Birds nest, grow, and learn to fly here. Bears stick to the deep forest and eat berries that grow in the shade.

Life is abundant here, protected by the mighty mountain. Yet, the mountain stands alone. It is a lonely mountain, tasked to protect this valley all on its own. When winter comes and it is covered with snow, the life around it seeks shelter, or else it is left out in the cold.

The lonely mountain continues to stand tall. Nothing can break its pride. It will protect the valley of life and forever be alone.

ON A SNOWY NIGHT

The first snow of the season begins to fall. The once green ground is now covered with a soft, fresh blanket of powder. The air has a chill to it. You are safe inside your warm, cozy house.

You watch the snow fall from the sky through your window and frozen rain floats elegantly down. No two snowflakes are alike. Each one is unique in the way it's formed, the way it falls to the ground, and the way it melts into a small, cool puddle.

A rocky chair waits by the window and a fire crackles softly. All you have to do is lean back and feel the warmth enveloping you. The chair rocks back and forth ever so slightly, with a gentle push.

The sky is dark but the snow seems to glow like tiny halos sitting atop the heads of tiny angels. The chair rocks you to sleep as the sound of the crackling fire soothes you. Sleep on this winter night and awake to a new world, covered in a fresh blanket of snow.

THE TORTOISE AND THE SNAIL

A tortoise is like a snail and a snail is like a tortoise. They both have so much in common, even if one is small while the other is a giant.

They both carry around a shell on their backs, acting not only as a home, but protection as well. They tend to crawl up inside their shells when they need to.

Neither of them can float in water or swim in it either. A snail will avoid water because it has no legs or arms to swim with. A tortoise stays clear of the water too because it would only sink to the bottom.

A tortoise and a snail would come in second in a race, because they both move too slow. Not that either of them would take a race, unless a rabbit happens to pass by.

The tortoise and the snail are so alike, yet they are neither friends nor family. They live far apart and never cross paths. Is it because they like different food or follow different dreams? No, I think it's simply because a snail is too small anda tortoise is too big.

THE LEAF ON THE LAKE

The large body of water lies still, like a mirror that holds the world's reflection. The world around it is just as still. The silence fills the air. Not even a whisper is heard in the stillness of the lake.

A single leaf is shaken loose from its hold on a tree by the soft, gentle breeze. It floats down, gracefully dancing through the air. The green leaf touches the still lake with a soft plop and sends ripple upon ripple through the waters.

One ripple after another travels from the center of the lake to the edge. The ripples build on each other. They're never-ending and somehow hypnotic.

The leaf remains in the center of the lake that is no longer still. It hovers on the surface, never sinking or fading. The lake resembles a tiny ocean and the ripples are its waves. They crash onto the shore, like a faint whisper.

One small leaf brings perfect stillness into perfect chaos. The smallest of things can make the largest impact.

THE FISH AND THE RIVER

The pristine water flows gently down the hill. It can only flow in this direction. The river curves and bends, falls and rises, slows and speeds up all the way to the end. It's like a rollercoaster.

This river is home to a special fish. The fish know they must swim with the river in order to reach what waits for them at the end. They must follow the flow of the water. They must glide through the slow parts, keep up through the fast parts, curve with the bends, and rise and fall where needed.

The river is kind to the fish and carries them safely down the hill, for the fish must make this journey every day. To the fish, the river has no end. It is never-ending and always flowing.

The river flows for us all but we must learn to flow with it, for fighting the current will get us nowhere.

A FIELD OF FLOWERS

An orange glow appears on the horizon, pushing through the dark, black sky. The night stars fight to shine bright, but the rising sun puts their light to shame. The field before you is sleeping, but with the glow of the sun comes the life hidden in the tall grass.

The field of flowers awakes underneath the warmth of the sun's glow, stretching their long green stems out, growing taller right before your eyes. They curl out their petals, exposing their pollen-filled center to the bright, enriching light.

They sleep for a long time, but now it is their time to shine. They breathe in the air, letting it filltheir lungs. They soak up the warmth, allowing itto brighten their colors. They stretch their roots deep into the dirt, gathering up all the nutrients they need for the day.

The field of flowers comes to life each day underneath the light of the rising sun.

A DEEP BREATH

Close your eyes and take a deep breath. As you breathe in you feel the cool air flowing down the back of your throat, filling your lungs. The air tastes sweet and smells fresh. It reminds you of a berry picked directly from the bush or a flower sitting in a vase of water just moments after being picked from the soil. That fresh smell surrounds you, and you feel refreshed.

Open your eyes and let the breath that has filled your lungs go. Release it into the air, and watchit flow away, rejoining the atmosphere. The fog surrounds you. You are made new with that one deep breath.

FLOATING THROUGH THE CLOUDS

The pure, white shine surrounds you as you float through the sky with a blanket of clouds beneath you. The wind flows through them, lifting subtle whiffs of mist from beneath the clouds into the sky above. The world below you turns slowly and the sky above opens up its doors.

The fluffy texture is unlike anything you have ever felt. A pillow filled with duck feathers and lined with silk would feel like a rock in comparison to the bed of clouds you now rest on.

They hold you up high—high above the sun, high above the stars, and high above the world. You are being carried toward the heavens. The doors open wide for you to come and go as you please. Lay still as you float through the clouds in your dreams.

ON THE WINGS OF A BUTTERFLY

Soar through the air. Dart from one flower to the next, only taking rest for a short moment before taking off again. The wings of a butterfly are simple yet elegant in their beauty. They carry the tiniest creature from one destination to the next. They never tire and they never require rest.

The wings of a butterfly are unique in every way. Like a snowflake, no two are alike. The butterfly is a rainbow of colors, or one solid color all the way through. It can have stripes or dots, or both if it chooses.

On the wings of a butterfly is where I'd like to be, to see all that they do and be where they have been.

A DROP OF DEW

The journey that is taken by a single drop of dew is like no other, and yet it is a journey taken each and every day. The sun is about to rise. The light from its warm glow can be seen in the orange-tinted, blue sky. The birds begin to chirp and their song is an indicator that the world is waking up.

A single drop of dew sits at the tip of a blade of grass. It is small compared to the world. Its life started just that morning, in the dim light of the stars, just before the sun awoke.

The sun begins its journey, rising into the morning sky. The dew drop falls slightly, flowing down the blade of grass. Nothing awaits it but a cold spot on the grass. Although it is small, it carriesgreat importance. Many are waiting for this dewdrop to complete its journey, many who crave itssweet, refreshing taste.

It shall end its journey on the ground as the sun's light fills the morning sky.

STANDING ON THE EDGE OF A CLIFF

You stand on the edge of a cliff, and a floor of clouds stretches out before you. You can't see the ground from where you are, but the sky is now close enough to touch. The sun is within an arm's reach and the stars float beside you.

It's as if you're standing on top of the world and you're far from the troubles that it brings. You could step out onto the clouds if you wanted to, but for now you remain at the edge.

The full moon sits at the horizon on your left while the sun occupies the horizon on your life. The sky is scattered by stars and clouds alike, and in the distance you see the glow of a rainbow.

It all looks like a painting made specially for you. You take a seat at the edge of the cliff as the day turns into night and the night turns into day. You sit and you wait for the painting to be complete.

FIREFLIES IN THE SKY

The world is silent. Silence has fallen and not a single sound can be heard. A mouse does not dare to squeak and an owl does not dare to hoot. There is only darkness and silence. In that silence a warm glow appears.

That glow is dim at first, like a lost ember from a fire that has since gone cold. The glow rises from the ground, fluttering like a petal in the wind, but there is no wind. This glow is soon joined by a second light, just as dim and small. A third light appears and a fourth light after that. They all glow and flutter as one.

The fireflies have come to life in the darkness and silence of the night. They spring from their slumbers and fly up into the sky. Their dim, warm glow burns like a blazing fire among the evening stars.

They rise up into the sky, posing as stars in the darkness. Their glow is a beacon to all, signaling that the night is alive and filled with wonder.

THE LONELY SNOWMAN

A fresh pile of snow is on the ground, rolled up into a ball, and stacked on top of three bigger balls. This snow is but a pile until formed into the shape of a man. All you need to do is add the features that turn it into a snowman.

You gather up pebbles. Theyare black andsmooth. You hold them up in your hand and notice they are as small and flat as a penny. These pebbles, if placed right, make up the snowman's gleaming eyes and pearly smile.

Now, you search the ground for a twig. Not just any twig, but a long, thin twig with a single end that splits into two on the other end. You find two of these and stick them into the side of the middle snowball, forming the arms of the snowman.

It's almost complete, all it needs is a hat and scarf to keep warm. It's now a fully formed snowman, but it's missing one thing: a friend. It's a lonely snowman standing where you built it.

A CANDLE IN THE WIND

Standing tall and proud, it doesn't bend in the wind. A candle stands on strong legs and holds itself up no matter what. When an idea sparks, a fire is born at the top of its head. The flame burns bright, a yellow glow that cannot reach far but still burns with a passion.

This flame is not as strong as the candle it sits on. The candle holds the flame as best it can, but it's made weaker by its heat. The candle begins to fade away, melting beneath the brilliant burn.

The flame is weak and bends easily. If a gust of wind were to blow, the flame would vanish even if the candle remained. It is a relationship where they need one another to be near, but at the same time they would be better off without the other there.

IN SEARCH OF FIREWOOD

Chop!
Chop!
Chop!

The sound echoes through the empty forest. It frightens away the birds, urging them to fly away from their nests. It spooks the rodents in the undergrowth, forcing them to run and hide.

A woodsman marches through the trees, swinging his axe about, chopping as he pleases. With each chop, a tree falls down. With each chop, the forest shakes. With each chop, he gathers firewood for the fire he wants to build that night.

A tree falls underneath his mighty axe and shakes the ground. He drags it away, up the hill to the cabin where he sleeps. He chops the fallen tree into smaller pieces, for a whole tree is far too big for his fire. As he chops away, the tree becomes smaller and the pile of fire logs beside it grows larger.

He drops his axe and retires to his bed, satisfied with the wood he has gathered for the day. Tonight he will build his fire and tomorrow he will return to the forest in search of more firewood.

ROASTING MARSHMALLOWS ON THE FIRE

Smoke rises through the air. Thin wisps of darkened clouds filled the open sky, twirling into indistinguishable patterns. Soft, orange embers are lifted up into the sky by the smoke and carried on the wind. They dance in the moonlight. Watch them twirl and glide as they leave the fire that brought them to life for the great unknown.

Hear the sizzle of the burning flame on the cold ground. Hear the hiss as the flames lap at the rocks surrounding it. Hear the cracking of the wood as the fire eats away at it, leaving nothing but bright, white coals burning hot.

The air is filled with a sweet smell as you hover over the fluffy, soft marshmallow over the flames. The flames reach up for the white treat and try to eat it, but you keep it safely away from its reach. Watch the white slowly brown all over as the sweet smell of roasted marshmallow rises to your nostrils. You know the taste is something the fire will envy you for.

A COZY MOLE HOLE

A hole in the ground is not a place you would find homely. You would not see it as being humble, neat, or cozy, but that is precisely how you would describe the hole of this particular mole.

This mole holds himself to a certain standard, and so he holds his hole to the same standards. His hole is a cozy one. The walls are smooth and decorated sparingly with art. The floor, which would genuinely be dirt, is covered with only the softest rugs for gentle feet. He has plenty of furniture, so that if you wanted a seat, you could have it. His furniture is all handmade and comfortable to say the least.

This hole is a cozy one and it is the hole of a mole who considered himself to be a gentleman.

A HOUSE FOR A MOUSE

How would you make a house for a mouse? It would need to be small, since mice are very small and would not like a house that is too big. It would need to be warm, since mice do not tolerate the cold well. It would need to be inviting, since mice have standards when it comes to those things. It would need to be humble, for a mouse is not one to boast or brag.

Making a house for a mouse is a small task, but it would be challenging. You would need a sturdy roof, in case it rains too hard. You would need thick walls to keep out the cold. You would need tiny furniture and measure it well, to make sure it fits just right. You would need a door of the perfect size, and don't forget the windows on all four sides.

Making a house for a mouse would be difficult indeed.

A CRACK IN THE EGG

An egg sits at the center of the nest that was made specially for it. The nest is wide enough for the egg to fit comfortably and the sides are high enough to stop it from rolling off.

The eggs shell is pristine, a musky white color witha certain glow and subtle dimples all throughout. It's a perfect dome, housing a small life that is about to begin. You know that this life is ready tobreak through when a small crack appears along the side of the egg.

The once pristine egg is no longer perfect, with a small crack marking its side. The crack issmall, but slowly it spreads out, becoming larger, spreading out into more, smaller cracks. The crack makes its way around the whole egg, forming its own pattern alongside the egg's dimple pattern.

The crack continues until life is able to burst from inside. Soon, the egg will be nothing more than shards of musky white on the ground, and a baby will take its first steps into the world.

THE ANIMALS ON THE FARM

The animals on the farm come in all different shapes and sizes. They each make their own sounds and play their own roles.

The chickens that live in the chicken coop eat their seeds and lay their eggs. The roosters crow loudly to wake up the farmer in the morning.

The cows live out in the field. They graze and eat the green grass all day, and sleep in the barn at night. In the morning, the farmer takes their milk to drink and sell.

The sheep stay in a herd and move as one. They make a lot of noise and eat a lot of grass, but the farmer needs their wool to make blankets in the winter.

There are many more animals to think of, each with their own purpose. The farmer cares for them all, as that is his job.

THE FROZEN LAKE

A lake that sits calmly, undisturbed by the world around it, makes for the world's clearest mirror. A still lake cannot be completely still. A gentle breeze or a falling leaf could disturb the waters, and when the waters are no longer still, the image becomes unclear.

The frozen lake does not worry about any of this. It sits undisturbed as the world continues around it. The wind may blow and the leaves may fall from the sky, but the frozen lake will remain still.

The frozen lake is a mirror for the whole world, and what you see in it can be only what is true. The frozen lake is filled with life, but like the water, this life is frozen. The fish that would swim freely through its waters are now frozen in time.

Soon, the waters will melt and life will continue. But until then, it remains frozen.

A SHORT WALK

The day is long and the road ahead of you is clear. The sun rises early in the morning. You place a pair of comfortable shoes on your feet and step outside your door.

The sun is high in the sky but it shines gently on your back. A cool breeze blows through your hair. You walk down the street on this quiet day. Not a single car is on the road, nor is there a soul to walk beside you.

The birds sing their songs, the crickets chirp in the grass, and the world turns around you. A short walk on a long day is all you need to clear your mind. Walk slow and take it all in, for the walk may be short but you have all the time in the world.

THE ROAR OF THE WIND

The world can show its dark side easily. There is a silence that cannot be broken when the world is at peace. Everything is still. This is a special time: when the world appears to be asleep.

There are also times when the world is the essence of chaos. Those are the times when the sky is dark and the clouds are angry, when lightning strikes the sky and thunder breaks the silence.

The world is filled with chaos, just on the verge of breaking through the peace and silence. The wind roars through the trees, bending them over and threatening to break them. The rain pours, slamming against the Earth.

This is a beautiful chaos that is needed to break the silence.

DANCING TREES

It's a wonder to see the trees dancing in the wind, to see their long, strong trunks bend and sway, to watch their branches wave back and forth, to see their leaves clinging on as they shake violently in the wind.

The crack of the trunk and the creak of the branches fills the air, but it's barely heard over the rustle of the leaves. The dance of the trees is one that can be long or it can be short. It entirely depends on the trees and how much they enjoy this dance.

The branches twirl around each other and the leaves join hands. Their song is one they sing on their own. They dance to their own music that we can only hear if we close our eyes.

A DAY IN THE GARDEN

The perfect day does not exist, but a day that is perfect for gardening does, and that day is today. The sun is out, but the thin wisp of a cloud glides over it, sheltering you from its intense heat and light.

The grass outside is green and soft to the touch. It's freshly cut, which means a sweet aroma fills the air. The garden is surrounded by a tall hedge, cut perfectly square. It shelters you from prying eyes and gives you your privacy.

You can sit on the grass and look up at the blue sky, as the white clouds float by, or you can sit on a garden chair and enjoy a cup of fresh juice in the open air. Perhaps a cup of tea and your pickof biscuits, too.

Sit here and listen to the sounds of nature fill your garden on this perfect gardening day.

THE ROCKING CHAIR

Sitting at the window is a rocking chair. It's not your rocking chair and you don't know how it got there, but it's waiting for you to come and sit down.

A rocking chair is reliable. It's comfortable and it makes you feel safe. You can rest in its grasp and never worry about the world disturbing the peace it wants to make for you.

With a slight rocking motion, back and forth, the rocking chair rocks you into a silent sleep. Back and forth it rocks, a subtle creak breaking the silence. Be still as the chair rocks away your fears and worries.

A SKY FILLED WITH STARS

The sky appears to be empty but it's not. The clouds are thick and hide from you what you do not know. You look up and search the empty sky for what you know to be there.

You look for the stars that light up the sky.They bring light to the darkness and life to the emptiness. They awake at night and sleep during the day. The stars shine each night even though they are not asked to. Without them, the world would be dark.

Looking up at the sky you know they'll always be there to shine brighter than any other light. You can rely on their glow and know they'll be there to pierce through the dark.

A COLD WINTER'S MORNING

Drip...drip...drip...

You awake to this sound on your windowsill early in the morning. You feel the cold in the air and on your nose and cheeks. You're kept safe and comfortable by the thick duvet that surrounds you.

You hear the dripping outside as the snow melts and trickles down your roof. The winter air wanders freely outside, but that air is kept at bay by the burning fire.

The crack and hiss of the fire lets you know that it's still lending its heat to you. You pull the duvet closer, pulling yourself snugly into its hold. You wrap yourself in its warmth and itis soft touch.

This winter morning can pass you by as you sleep, protected in this safe place.

THE BUZZING BEE IS A BUSY BEE

The buzzing of a bee lets you know that they are busy. They are busy flying from one flower to the next. They are busy collecting pollen. They are busy making honey. A bee is the busiest bug out there.

A bee buzzes as it takes wing, leaving the hive and setting out into the world. It buzzes as it lands on a flower, grabbing as much pollen as it can before flying to the next. It buzzes as it turns that pollen into honey, a sweet treat for others to eat.

The buzzing bee is the busiest bee of all, so make sure you never get in the way of a bee as it buzzes on by.

THE SLEEPY OWL

Asleep in its hole, an owl is not to be disturbed. It's a creature of habit, and its habit is to sleep when the sun is high in the sky. A hole in a tree is where you'll find an owl, deep in its sleep.

How can we tell if an owl dreams? Does an owl toss and turn in its sleep. Does it hoot silently when no one is there to hear? If you tiptoe through the forest and peek into the holes in a tree you might find a sleepy owl waiting.

If you go looking for an owl in its sleep, be careful not to wake it. The day may belong to you but the night is what the owl waits for. During the day the owl sleeps but at night the owl comes to life and soars through the sky.

Let it sleep for now, because a sleepy owl cannot soar through the sky.

MORNING MIST

It's a special kind of morning. The air is still, the clouds in the sky are thick, and although the sun is beginning to rise, it's hidden from our eyes. This is a morning where mist covers the ground.

The mist seems to roll in from nowhere yet everywhere. The dew on the grass and moisture in the air rise up, like steam. The heat from the sun is piercing through the clouds, but the sun's light is still blocked behind them.

You wade through the morning mist as if wading through a still lake—it's so thick that you cannot disturb its flow. It exists around you. You exist alongside it. Once the sky clears and the sun shines, the mist will be gone.

SITTING IN THE SHADE OF A TREE

A tree stands tall above the world. It's stature is great and its shadow is long. Its branches stretch out far and wide, like the limbs of a giant. Its leaves are large and glow with a bright green color.

This tree is a giant among trees, but it stands alone in a field of grass. Nothing stands beside it and no one challenges its claim.

When the sun shines and the heat is too much to bear, this tree provides shade for those who ask for it. If you wander past, you may take a moment to sit down in its shade. This shade is your protection from the heat.

The tree will continue to stand tall until the end of its days and it will provide shade to those who are willing to sit and stay a while.

HOT CHOCOLATE IN THE SNOW

The snow drifts down from the sky. The clouds are filled with water and the air is cold enough to freeze the droplets. As the snow slowly floats towards the ground, the world begins to change. Winter has come, and the world seems a little darker without the sun.

Still, the snow appears to glow. It has a light of its own and it brightens the winter day. It's white glow and the cold air make a perfect atmosphere for a hot cup of cocoa.

With your hot chocolate in hand you step out into the cold, winter air. Steam rises from your cup and fog rides on your breath. You are surrounded by the cold, but the hot chocolate in your hands keeps you warm.

Drink its sweetness as the snow falls around you. Feel the warmth through your body and allow your soul to glide with the flakes of snow.

SIZZLING BACON

Waking up in the morning can be hard. You sink into your bed, for you would not want to leave its warm embrace. Still, you cannot sleep the day away.

The sound of hissing fills your ears, and the smell of bacon grabs your attention. Bacon sizzles in a pan with eggs. Toast pops up out of the toaster and the kettle whistles for your tea.

It's the perfect breakfast to help you get up in the morning. It's a breakfast to lure you out of bed and fill you with energy for the day. The sound of sizzling bacon is all you need to hear to knowyour breakfast is waiting for you to get out of bed.

ROLLING IN THE GRASS

To be a kid again would be wonderful. To play all day in the sun, not worrying about the dirt onyour clothes or the leaves in your hair. You have nothing to do and nowhere to be. There's no one to look at you funny when you roll down a hill.

You can go roll in the grass, run through a field, climb up a tree, jump into a puddle, and eat whatever food you want to eat. You don't need to worry about anything. To be a kid again would be great.

Children are children, and it's as simple as that.It doesn't matter what they do, it's normal for a child to do whatever they want. For one day, let out the child within you. Don't hide them away; let them come out and play. No one is looking and no one cares. For one day, be a child again.

THE TEA PARTY IN THE WOODS

The woods is a funny place to have a tea party, buta tea party in the woods awaits you. Walk downthe path laid out before you. It's hard to miss. It'sthe only path through the woods and it's the only path that will lead you to the tea party.

The path curves and winds, but it will take you where you need to be. The tea party will be fun. There will be tea and cakes and games to play. Many animals will come and join you throughout the day.

The birds love to sip on tea and the bees will love to eat the sugar. The squirrels will hog the cake and the bunnies will eat all of the muffins. There'll be plenty left for you as long as you get there on time.

A tea party in the woods will be a great way to spend the day.

THE RED ROSE AND THE WHITE ROSE

The red rose and the white rose each sit on a wall. The red rose faces the west while the white rose faces the east. The red rose does not care for the white rose and the white rose does not care for the red rose.

The white rose envies the red rose, for its deep color. The red rose envies the white rose for its splendid glow. The white rose does not care much for its lack of color and the red rose wishes it could glow in the light.

It does neither good to envy the other, for the beauty they share can be seen by all but themselves. The shape of a rose is unlike any other. It's natural and gracious. The white rose and the red rose are more alike than they think.

READING BY THE LAKE

Sit down on the wet grass and lean back against the trunk of a tree. Feel the cool breeze blow through your hair and smell the sweetness in the fresh air. Today is the perfect day to read by the lake.

The water is calm with slight ripples forming at the center of the lake, moving towards the edges. Your book lays open on your lap. The pages are filled with words you wish to read or images you want to see. The story tells itself.

Sit back and let the story unfold in front of you while the lake remains still beside you. Reading by the lake is the perfect way to spend this perfect day.

A HOUSE MADE OF FLOWERS

Deep in the forest, hidden by those who don't understand, is a house made entirely of flowers. This house stands empty, for no one can live in it. It's there only for travelers who wish to rest their feet and stay for the night.

The roof is lined with dandelions, their white petals and yellow centers catching the sun and shining bright. The windows are open, lined with twine that has been twisted and shaped. The walls are made of roses of every shape, size, and color, and the door is made of violets.

The flowers hold themselves together with their stems and cling tightly together. The wind or rain cannot pull them apart. This house made of flowers is here to stay. Come inside and spend the night, because its door is open to any traveler who wanders by.

THE SMALL PEOPLE

The small people are all around us. They sneak under our feet and hide from our sight. They're small enough to squeeze through a mouse hole and dance on the palm of our hands.

The small people want what we don't. They take unwanted things and use them. Your lost sock makes a cozy blanket or a nice rug. Your missing earring holds up the window in their house.

If something disappears you can be sure the small people have it. They need it more than us, so we cannot be mad at them for taking it. The small people are all around us. We live in peace with them as long as they stay hidden.

WILDFIRE

A fire burns with a passion. It's hungry and angry. A fire eats endlessly, never becoming full. It sucks up the air and eats everything in sight, justto grow larger and burn hotter.

A wildfire cannot be stopped. It burns and consumes all in its path. A wildfire burns through the world, turning trees to ash and flowers to embers. It's smoke fills the air and its orange glow lights up the darkened sky.

It's hiss turns into a roar and its flames bite hard. It is a wild animal: untameable and uncontrollable. Water is its only enemy and chaos is its true friend. Feed the fire if you dare, but beware the monster hiding within.

A PIG CAN'T LOOK UP

A pig is a simple creature. It's small and round. It has a long snout for sniffing and a big mouth for eating. It has short legs and a short neck. This short neck is why a pig cannot look up to the sky.

A pig can roll around in the mud and run around. A pig can jump up and down or even dance. A pig knows how to look down or even left and right, but a pig cannot look up even if they try.

The sky is a thing a pig has never seen, unless it lies on its back and looks down towards its round belly. The stars shine bright but the pig does not see them twinkling. The moon glows in the dark but the pig cannot look at its luminosity. The birds fly past but the pig doesn't doesn't see their feathers fall to the ground.

The sky is a mystery, and a part of the unknown for a pig who cannot look up.

A CROCODILE'S TONGUE

A crocodile has a long nose and a short tongue. It's teeth are long and sharp, and its jaw snaps down hard. What happens when a crocodile bites its tongue? It can't, because a crocodile can't stick out its tongue.

Kids stick their tongues out to tease and we stick our tongues out to eat ice cream. We stick our tongues out when we're being silly or having fun, and we stick our tongues out to taste the falling rain.

We stick our tongues out because we can, but a crocodile simply can't. Its tongue is far too short and its nose is far too long. It's a good thing it can't, because a crocodile might accidently bite off its poor tongue.

A TIGER'S STRIPES

A tiger is known for its black stripes. Without its stripes, what would a tiger be? If a tiger was born with no fur, would it still be a tiger at all? Yes, it would, because a tiger's stripes are on its skin, not its fur.

A tiger is a proud and strong creature. They are the noble princes of nature. Their stripes represent nobility and make them distinguished. The gentle tiger wears its stripes on its skin so it can never be mistaken for anything other than what it is.

A tiger's stripes are what make the tiger, so nature has made sure they will always wear them. Try to shave a tiger if you can, but even then they will still display the stripes that make it a tiger.

A GIANT SQUID'S EYES

A giant squid floats about in the ocean, swimming deep down where no one else dares to go. The deepest and darkest part of the ocean is what the giant squid calls home.

A giant squid's eyes are the largest eyes on the planet, but it does not use them to see. What is there to see in the deepest and darkest part of the ocean, where the squid chooses to be?

The ocean is large and there's plenty of space to swim, but the giant squid chooses to swim where no one else can venture. It's too dark to see, so its giant eyes remain unused. If only it could see through the dark, or if it glowed whenever it looked around.

The giant squid's eyes have to stay closed, until they choose to swim up where they can actually see, but then the world will be able to see them, and that would not end well for the squid you see.

A CAT THAT DOESN'T BITE

Have you met the cat that doesn't bite or the cat that doesn't scratch? Have you seen the cat with no fur or the cat with no claws? Do you know the cat that cannot meow or the cat that refuses to purr?

These cats all live together in a big house covered with fur. They lay around, doing nothing all day. What is a cat to do except do cat things?

Cats are supposed to bite and they are meant to scratch. A cat is expected to have claws and fur. Cats usually like to meow and purr. If a cat doesn't do any of these things, is it still a cat?

These cats live in their house because there is nowhere else to go. There isn't a place in this world for a cat who does not want to be a cat. Instead, they live here and do what they want to do, which has nothing to do with being a cat at all.

BIRDS TAKING FLIGHT

How can a bird spread its wings and take flight? Is it something they learn or is it somethingthat comes naturally? Can they dance and sing if they are not taught, or are they born with the knowledge they need to do it all?

A bird can spread its wings and leap from the nest. There is nothing to stop it from falling straight down to the ground. The wind beneath their wings keeps them in the air.

A bird takes flight without ever even knowing if the wind will keep them afloat or let them fall down. They leap from their nests and flap their wings. It trusts in itself to not fall. It knows that if it has wings it must be able to fly.

A PENGUIN IN A SUIT

A penguin does not wear a suit, although it looks as if it does. The penguin does not wear clothes, even if the place it lives in is cold. If a penguin was to wear a suit, it would be a funny sight, one that I'm sure would have us all laughing with delight.

A penguin's skin is made of black and white. It is a gentleman in disguise. It walks with its head held high and its flippers at its sides. It bows to say hello and goodbye. A penguin in a suit would be a sight indeed, but not a shocking one I do believe.

Perhaps one day a penguin will agree to wear a suit for us all to see. I believe a penguin is a true gentleman and a suit was made to be worn by this creature. We have to wait and see.

THE DONKEY AND THE HORSE

A donkey once walked by a horse grazing in a wide, open field. The donkey smiled and greeted him, but the horse turned his nose up at the donkey.

"I cannot talk to you," the horse said. "You are a donkey."

"I don't understand," said the donkey. "What is wrong with me being a donkey?"

"A donkey and a horse cannot speak. We are simply too different."

"How are we different?" the donkey asked.

The donkey saw how they both had four legs and a tail. They both ate grass and they both liked to walk around. The donkey had hair on its head, as did the horse. They each had two eyes, two ears, and a long nose on the front of their face.

To the donkey there was no difference between him and the horse. He simply didn't understand. The horse shook his head because he did not understand himself, but he believed himself to be better, and that will never change.

THE NINE-TAILED FOX

The fox with nine tails is but a myth or a legend to most. It is a fox with fur as orange as a blazing fire and eyes as blue as the clear sky. Its teeth are sharp as knives and white as snow. It's claws are long and deadly, but never used unless necessary. It has not one, but nine tails.

This fox is known to many as either a good omen or a bad one. If you see this fox with nine tails out in the world, you may have something good coming to you, but if you spot it stalking you in the dark, be aware that bad things are soon to follow.

Do not worry, for the nine-tailed fox has not yet been seen. It is a myth and a legend not to be taken seriously. If you do ever spot it out and about, take your time, for its beauty is unlike anything you'll ever see.

THE WONDERFUL AND WILD OCEAN

The ocean is filled with many wonders and delights, but it also holds many fears and frights.

The blue whale is beautiful and majestic. The crab is silly and fun. The clown fish does not tell jokes, but its bright colors are a sight to behold. Shrimp are small and tasty, and oysters can be eaten or used for their pearls.

All this beauty and fun can be found in the ocean—wonderful and wild—but terror and fearful sights can be found too: The shark, with its teeth sharp and its appetite large. The octopus is dangerous indeed, with eight arms and plenty of black ink. The eel gives us quite a shock, and the snakes slither down there too.

The ocean is no place for us to swim. It's wonderful and wild, and it's meant for the animals to roam.

RAISE A TOAST

We raise a toast to celebrate. When there is good news to hear or an achievement to celebrate, we raise our glasses and toast to it. Why do we do this?

In ancient Rome it was believed that a piece of toast in your glass of wine was a symbol of good health. When you raise your glass you raise a toast. We no longer place toast in our wine, but the saying is still the same.

Next time someone says, "Raise a toast," make sure to check your glasses. You wouldn't want to sip your wine only to find a piece of toast floating about. It is meant for your good health, but wine-soaked toast can't taste all that good.

A BLUE LOBSTER

A lobster is usually red. This is the norm. When you see a lobster you often see its deep, red shell. Lobsters are not known for being any other color. But what of the blue lobster?

The blue lobster does exist, but it is said that only 1 in 2 million lobsters are blue. That is truly rareand a wonder. Know that if you ever see a blue lobster that it is the 1 out of 2 million lobsters to be born with a blue color.

The lobster does not know how rare and special it is. Would a blue lobster even know that it is blue? Does a red lobster look at it and laugh? No,I think a blue lobster sees itself and knows that it is rare.

A SHRIMP'S HEART IS IN ITS HEAD

Where is your heart? Is it in your chest? Does your heart beat loud enough for you to hear? Can you feel the heartbeat through your chest? Your heart beats in your chest, but for a shrimp, its heart is in its head.

A shrimp can think or it can feel. It has to do both since its heart and brain share the same space. Can you imagine if your mind and heart were to be so close? They would argue over every little thing you did.

The heart and mind are very different. The heart thinks only of what it wants but the mind thinks of what it needs. Nothing could be more different than a heart and a mind, but for a shrimp, its heart is its mind.

THE SQUIRREL THAT LOST ITS NUTS

Scurrying around the forest floor and climbing up the trunks of trees, the squirrel is one of the busiest creatures indeed.

A squirrel searches all day for food. They search on the ground and they search through the trees. They look for berries and they search for grapes, but what they hope to find is nuts.

A squirrel craves nuts and searches day and night for them. One problem a squirrel encounters though, is that they tend to lose the nuts they find. If a squirrel finds a nut, they'll bury the nut for safe keeping, but they're so silly that they forget where they buried the nut.

That nut will lay in the ground, where nature will care for it, and soon it will grow into a tree. The squirrel will find another nut and they might keep this one, but the ones that they forget will soon be majestic trees.

THE FOREST OF GIANTS

If you come across the forest of giants, what would you do? Would you walk around it or just go straight through? There is no path that can lead you to the other side, but there are plenty of creatures to ask along the way.

You could ask the rabbit which way to go, but he'll give you directions through his tunnels. The birds could show you the way, but you might lose them above the canopy of trees. If you ask the snail he'd be happy to show you the way, but he travels slower than most other creatures would.

The forest of giants is a place you need to see, but traveling through it might be a difficult task.

THE MUSHROOM HOUSE

Somewhere on the ground you may find a little mushroom house. It's like any other house, although it's mostly made of mushrooms. It has a door, with a beautiful bronze door handle. It has windows, with lovely window sills made from twisted vines.

There is a tiny cobblestone pathway that leads up to the mushroom house and a lovely garden of the tiniest flowers surrounds it.

Who lives in this mushroom house? We don't know. It could be a snail, or an ant, or a tiny person. It's a lovely home for anyone to live in.

WHEN DOGS RUN

When a dog runs it's entirely impossible to stop them. They can run for days, if they are running in the right direction. There's nothing they love to do more. If a dog could run forever, where wouldthey go?

Would they run across fields of grass and through puddles of mud? Would they run through a meat store and take all the sausages they can grab? Would they not care about where they run too?

I think if a dog could run forever, they would run straight back to you.

THE TINIEST BOAT

The tiniest boat sails on the tiniest sea. If a sea were tiny, how small would it be to you and me? It would be smaller than a puddle. Perhaps it would be only the size of a drop. If the sea is smaller than a drop, how small is the boat that sails on it?

The tiniest boat sails towards the tiniest piece of land—a small piece of rock with just a bit of sand. It's no bigger than the tip of your pinky, but it's got palm trees, coconuts, and starfish aplenty.

The tiniest boat sailing on the tiniest sea, could not be seen by either you or me.

THE CURIOUS FISH

The tail of the curious fish is a sad one indeed, for the fish lost its tail you see. The tail swam too close to shore, for it wanted to see what was going on where the people walked.

One day the fish thought he saw something strange. A creature that walked on all fours anda tail trailing behind it. The fish swam up close to see, for it had not seen anything like it before.

When the fish got close, the creature grabbed it. It's a cat and it had him. The fish swam as hard as he could and got away, but the cat had taken his tail and ate it whole.

THE DOOR IN THE TREE

There stands a single tree in the center of a wide, open field. No one knows who planted the tree or how it came to be there. If you walk just a little closer, you'll notice something strange.

This is something that you wouldn't think to see on a tree. It's the oddest thing indeed. You walk around and you see a door, right in the middle of the tree trunk.

You try the door handle, but it's locked. You decide to knock, but no one answers. A door in a tree... Who would have thought? Is it an entrance or an exit? Does someone live inside the tree, or is there somewhere else it leads?

A SHIP IN A BOTTLE

There is a ship in a bottle, trapped for all eternity. The sailor that sails it is trapped there too. He can't do much from his prison, but when he was on the sea he was relentless.

He was a pirate, seeking treasure and stealing gold. He was ruthless and deadly, a menace to the oceans and an enemy to many.

He crossed a gypsy once and one should never do that. He stole the gypsy's heart and so she trapped him in a bottle. She'll keep him for all eternity, or until he returns her heart.

SHAPES IN THE CLOUDS

Lay down on the ground and make some shapes in the sky. The clouds are thick and there are many. They float gently by, going from the left to the right. Watch them come close and you will see shapes appear where none should be: A cat playing with a ball of yarn to the left, and a goldfish in a bowl to the right. They cross each other and now the cat is playing with the goldfish's bowl. A crocodile in a top hat, and an onion with a moustache. A rabbit with a walking stick, and a juggling mouse. Dancing nuts, gossiping grapes, twisty trees, and singing flowers, to name a few.

Clouds take many funny shapes. Wouldn't you agree?

THE MOVING MOUNTAIN

How does a mountain move? For a thing so large to move without anyone noticing, how could it be? The mountain does move indeed.

Every year it gets a little short or it seems a little further away. The mountain does move but it has mastered the art of moving slowly.

The mountain moves, but when it does move it does it so slowly that it appears as if it's standing still. If you ever think a mountain is moving, but you cannot see because the mountain is just moving slowly.

NINE LIVES

A cat has nine lives, but what does he do with them?

Can a cat spend one life on the streets, exploring every alleyway, going on an adventure every day? Can he then spend the next life indoors, lazing about all day, being fed the finest food and sleeping in a warm bed?

A cat may spend all nine lives how he wishes. As long as each life is as long as can be, a cat can spend all nine however he pleases.

KINGS AND QUEENS

Kings, queens, and jokers are all lined up nicely. Which one will go first, to be placed face-up and smiling? It's a game of cards you see, and only one can be the winner.

The king is ready to bow his head, show off his crown, and prove he is the best. The queen shall show off her beauty, wave her hand, and take home the winner's crown. The joker is sneaky and knows very well that he will be the winning clown.

The joker steps forward, placing his hands on his hips. He won. It was no competition. How can the king and queen compete if they have no heads?

SANDCASTLE

The sandcastle stands on its own, surrounded by piles of stone. No other sandcastles exist in this place. Just this one sandcastle, in its own space.

The sand was brought here on its own and pulled together in this place of stone. The castle was born and around it looked. It saw nothing. No one. Not a thing.

There was a bucket, in the hands of a child, which was used to bring more sand out here to the wilds. Will the sand be for another castle or perhaps for something else completely? Let's hope the sand castle won't be alone for eternity.

STARFISH AND SAND ANGLES

A starfish cannot walk on land, nor can it fly. It lives in the ocean but it doesn't know how to swim or dive. A starfish is all arms, five in total. It has no fins, legs, or wings that can be useful.

A starfish once wandered onto the land and wanted to make a snow angel, but one that was made of sand—a sand angel. It laid down flat and spread out its arms. It waved them up and down and smiled the whole time.

When the starfish got up to look at its work it realized it had far too many arms to make a sand angel.

THE WISHING STAR

Up in the night sky, if you look, you'll see millions of bright lights shining as bright as can be. These are stars or fireflies that got stuck in the sky. They shine brightly just for you and me.

There is one star among them, more specialthan the rest. It has a special power that none ofthem can match. It's the wishing star, and it does precisely that. Wish upon it and what you wish for you shall have.

Search the skies and hope that you find the wishing star wherever it may hide. When you find it, make sure to close your eyes. Wish upon it and you'll receive what you desire.

THE GIRL WITH LONG HAIR

A little girl who is only as tall as a goat, has the longest hair. It stretches down her back and far past her ankles. It drags along the floor when she walks.

Sometimes she trips on it and falls over. Others have to stumble around her hair and try not to step on it. Her hair is dirty, filled with dirt and twigs. She finds it hard to brush, as her arms are far too short.

One night, while she sleeps, a man snuck into her house and cut her hair. He cut it all off, everylast strand. Still she sleeps and doesn't wake up again.

Her hair was her life, and she had lived for so long. Without her hair, she cannot wake up at all.

THE MOUSE WITH THE CLOCK

A mouse rushed out of his house early in the morning. He ran so fast that no one could even say hello. He was late, you see, and how did he know? Because of the watch he kept in his home.

The watch was far too big for him to carry around. It was clunky and it made an awfully loud sound. He kept and leaned it against a wall. Now he always knew the time of day.

The mouse was late, and the clock told himthis. What he was late for no one could really understand. Becausethere was nothingimportant for a mouse to do. He was just a mouse after all.

THE LOST ICE

The ice used to live inside the freezer and it thought it was quite nice. It was always cold and always dark, and this was the life he liked.

One day the freezer opened and let the light in. He shut his eyes tight and hoped it would end. He felt something grab hold of him and lift him up. This was just his luck.

He left the freezer behind and felt the warmth around him. This was no good at all, he thought. He needed it to be colder. He struggled and wiggled until at last, whatever was holding him, lost its grasp.

He fell down to the floor and bounced away. The ice became lost and never found its way back to the freezer again.

CONCLUSION

Look at the world around you and notice everything. Notice the sound of the wind as it rushes past your ears. Notice the smell of the freshly cut grass of the rain hidden in the clouds. Feel the heat of the sun or the cold of the moon.

Stimulate your mind and keep it active. These stories show you the wonders of the world and the stretch of the imagination. Don't stop wondering and don't stop imagining.

Stop and notice the world in order to keep your mind active, and use all of your senses to stimulate your memory. The world around you is the only story book you need and it has many tales to tell.

Printed in Great Britain
by Amazon

37122018R00066